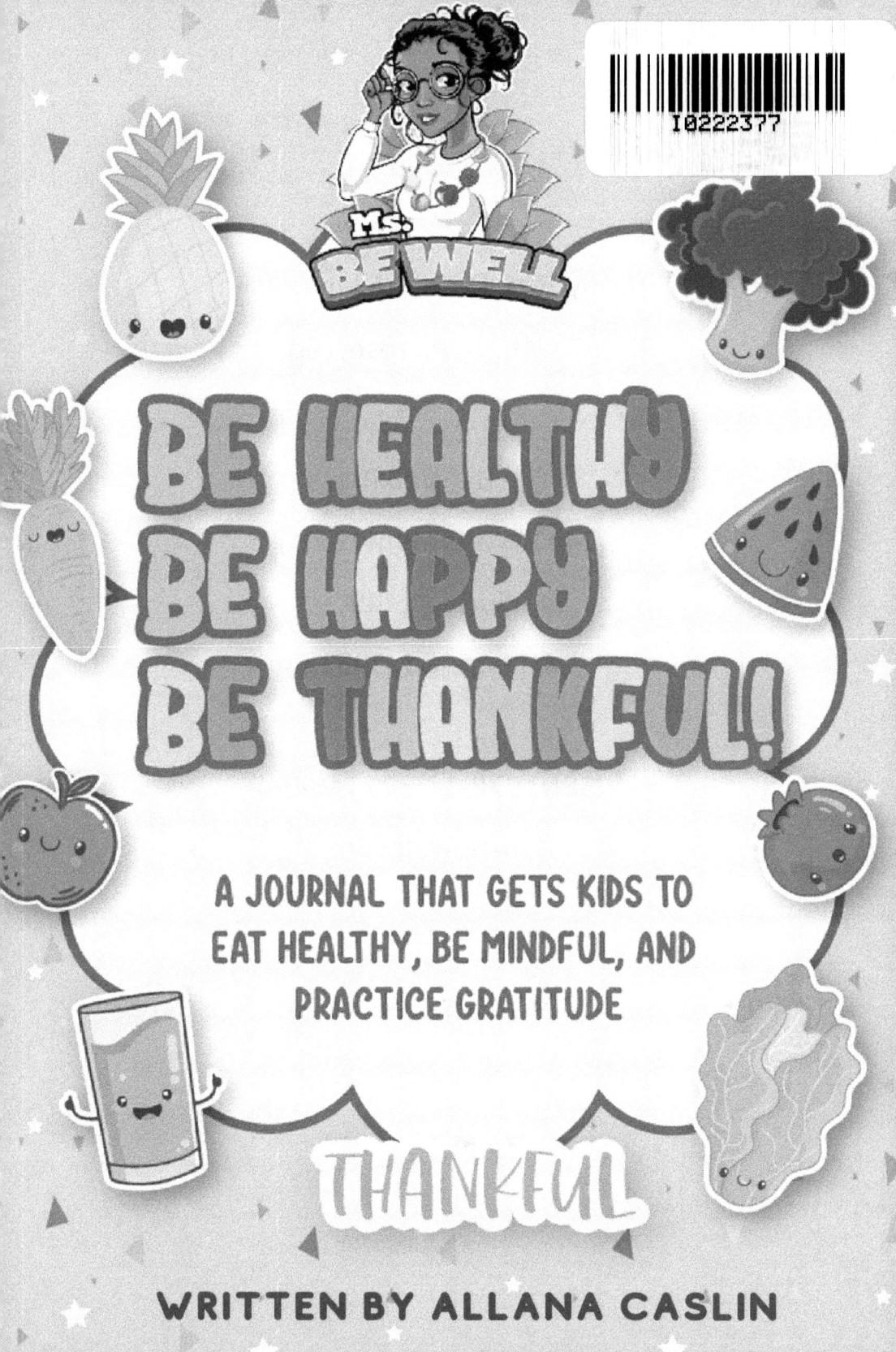

Copyright © 2021 Allana Caslin

All rights reserved.

The Be Well Press

1441 Woodmont Ln NW

Suite #1449

Atlanta, Ga. 30318

ISBN: 978-1-7371146-0-4

msbewell.com

Why do many adults struggle with keeping good habits? Because they don't form them when they're young. Studies show that teaching kids positive behaviors during childhood can set them up with healthy habits for life! "Be Healthy Be Happy Be Thankful!" is the perfect recipe for cultivating a lifestyle of mindfulness, healthy habits, and gratitude in young people.

As a certified Health & Physical Education teacher and the creator of the "Ms. Be Well" wellness character it's been my mission to instill the value of developing healthy lifestyle choices in young people. This daily journal is a tool to create the habits that can serve them for a lifetime.

In just 3 minutes a day young people can take ownership of their journey by acknowledging their feelings and what makes them happy, tracking their healthy habits (fruit, veggie, and water consumption) and focusing on the things they are grateful for.

The journey to transform a young person into their healthier, happier, and more grateful self, starts here!

For more from Ms. Be Well visit msbewell.com!

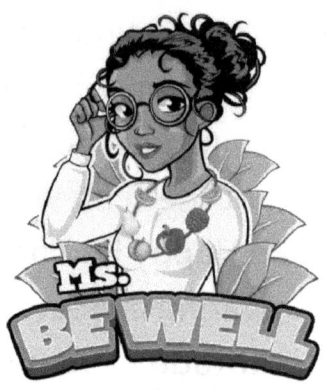

THIS BOOK BELONGS TO

_____

_____

TODAY

Date: Sun Mon Tues Weds Thurs Fri Sat ___ / ___ / ___

I Feel... ☺ ☺   😐 ☹ ☹

I AM HEALTHY!

What Fruits and Veggies Did I Eat?

_____
_____
_____

How Much Water Did I Drink?

🥛 🥛 🥛 🥛 🥛 🥛 🥛 🥛

I AM HAPPY!

What Made Me Feel Happy Today?

_____
_____
_____

I AM THANKFUL!

I Am Thankful For...

_____
_____
_____

TODAY

Date: Sun Mon Tues Weds Thurs Fri Sat ___/___/___

I Feel...   ☺   ☺   😐   ☹   ☹

I AM HEALTHY!

What Fruits and Veggies Did I Eat?

_____
_____
_____

How Much Water Did I Drink?

🥛 🥛 🥛 🥛 🥛 🥛 🥛 🥛

I AM HAPPY!

What Made Me Feel Happy Today?

_____
_____
_____

I AM THANKFUL!

I Am Thankful For...

_____
_____
_____

TODAY

Date: Sun   Mon   Tues   Weds   Thurs   Fri   Sat ___ / ___ / ___

I Feel...   ☺   ☺   ☺   ☹   ☹

I AM HEALTHY!

What Fruits and Veggies Did I Eat?

_____
_____
_____

How Much Water Did I Drink?

🥛 🥛 🥛 🥛 🥛 🥛 🥛 🥛

I AM HAPPY!

What Made Me Feel Happy Today?

_____
_____
_____

I AM THANKFUL!

I Am Thankful For...

_____
_____
_____

TODAY

Date: Sun Mon Tues Weds Thurs Fri Sat ___/___/___

I Feel...   ☺   ☺   😐   ☹   ☹

I AM HEALTHY!

What Fruits and Veggies Did I Eat?

_____
_____
_____

How Much Water Did I Drink?

I AM HAPPY!

What Made Me Feel Happy Today?

_____
_____
_____

I AM THANKFUL!

I Am Thankful For...

_____
_____
_____

TODAY

Date: Sun Mon Tues Weds Thurs Fri Sat ___/___/___

I Feel... ☺ ☺   😐 ☹ ☹

I AM HEALTHY!

What Fruits and Veggies Did I Eat?

_____
_____
_____

How Much Water Did I Drink?

🥛 🥛 🥛 🥛 🥛 🥛 🥛 🥛

I AM HAPPY!

What Made Me Feel Happy Today?

_____
_____
_____

I AM THANKFUL!

I Am Thankful For...

_____
_____
_____

TODAY

Date: Sun Mon Tues Weds Thurs Fri Sat ___/___/___

I Feel... ☺ ☺   😐 ☹ ☹

I AM HEALTHY!

What Fruits and Veggies Did I Eat?

_____
_____
_____

How Much Water Did I Drink?

🥛 🥛 🥛 🥛 🥛 🥛 🥛 🥛

I AM HAPPY!

What Made Me Feel Happy Today?

_____
_____
_____

I AM THANKFUL!

I Am Thankful For...

_____
_____
_____

TODAY

Date: Sun Mon Tues Weds Thurs Fri Sat ___/___/___

I Feel... ☺ ☺ 😐 ☹ ☹

I AM HEALTHY!

What Fruits and Veggies Did I Eat?

_____
_____
_____

How Much Water Did I Drink?

🥛 🥛 🥛 🥛 🥛 🥛 🥛 🥛

I AM HAPPY!

What Made Me Feel Happy Today?

_____
_____
_____

I AM THANKFUL!

I Am Thankful For...

_____
_____
_____

TODAY

Date: Sun Mon Tues Weds Thurs Fri Sat ___/___/___

I Feel...   ☺   ☺   😐   ☹   ☹

I AM HEALTHY!

What Fruits and Veggies Did I Eat?

_____
_____
_____

How Much Water Did I Drink?

I AM HAPPY!

What Made Me Feel Happy Today?

_____
_____
_____

I AM THANKFUL!

I Am Thankful For...

_____
_____
_____

TODAY

Date: Sun Mon Tues Weds Thurs Fri Sat ___/___/___

I Feel... ☺ ☺   😐 ☹ ☹

I AM HEALTHY!

What Fruits and Veggies Did I Eat?

_____
_____
_____

How Much Water Did I Drink?

🥛 🥛 🥛 🥛 🥛 🥛 🥛 🥛

I AM HAPPY!

What Made Me Feel Happy Today?

_____
_____
_____

I AM THANKFUL!

I Am Thankful For...

_____
_____
_____

TODAY

Date: Sun Mon Tues Weds Thurs Fri Sat ___/___/___

I Feel... ☺ ☺ ☺ ☹ ☹

I AM HEALTHY!

What Fruits and Veggies Did I Eat?

_____
_____
_____

How Much Water Did I Drink?

I AM HAPPY!

What Made Me Feel Happy Today?

_____
_____
_____

I AM THANKFUL!

I Am Thankful For...

_____
_____
_____

TODAY

Date: Sun Mon Tues Weds Thurs Fri Sat ___/___/___

I Feel...   ☺   ☺   😐   ☹   ☹

I AM HEALTHY!

What Fruits and Veggies Did I Eat?

_____
_____
_____

How Much Water Did I Drink?

🥛 🥛 🥛 🥛 🥛 🥛 🥛 🥛

I AM HAPPY!

What Made Me Feel Happy Today?

_____
_____
_____

I AM THANKFUL!

I Am Thankful For...

_____
_____
_____

TODAY

Date: Sun   Mon   Tues   Weds   Thurs   Fri   Sat ___ /___ /___

I Feel...   ☺   ☺   ☺   ☹   ☹

I AM HEALTHY!

What Fruits and Veggies Did I Eat?

_____
_____
_____

How Much Water Did I Drink?

🥛 🥛 🥛 🥛 🥛 🥛 🥛 🥛

I AM HAPPY!

What Made Me Feel Happy Today?

_____
_____
_____

I AM THANKFUL!

I Am Thankful For...

_____
_____
_____

TODAY

Date: Sun Mon Tues Weds Thurs Fri Sat ___/___/___

I Feel...   ☺   ☺   😐   ☹   ☹

I AM HEALTHY!

What Fruits and Veggies Did I Eat?
_____
_____
_____

How Much Water Did I Drink?

🥛 🥛 🥛 🥛 🥛 🥛 🥛 🥛

I AM HAPPY!

What Made Me Feel Happy Today?
_____
_____
_____

I AM THANKFUL!

I Am Thankful For...
_____
_____
_____

TODAY

Date: Sun Mon Tues Weds Thurs Fri Sat ___/___/___

I Feel... ☺ ☺ 😐 ☹ ☹

I AM HEALTHY!

What Fruits and Veggies Did I Eat?

_____
_____
_____

How Much Water Did I Drink?

I AM HAPPY!

What Made Me Feel Happy Today?

_____
_____
_____

I AM THANKFUL!

I Am Thankful For...

_____
_____
_____

TODAY

Date: Sun Mon Tues Weds Thurs Fri Sat ___/___/___

I Feel... ☺ ☺   😐 ☹ ☹

I AM HEALTHY!

What Fruits and Veggies Did I Eat?

_____
_____
_____

How Much Water Did I Drink?

🥛 🥛 🥛 🥛 🥛 🥛 🥛 🥛

I AM HAPPY!

What Made Me Feel Happy Today?

_____
_____
_____

I AM THANKFUL!

I Am Thankful For...

_____
_____
_____

TODAY

Date: Sun Mon Tues Weds Thurs Fri Sat ___/___/___

I Feel... ☺ ☺ ☺ ☹ ☹

I AM HEALTHY!

What Fruits and Veggies Did I Eat?

_____
_____
_____

How Much Water Did I Drink?

🥛 🥛 🥛 🥛 🥛 🥛 🥛 🥛

I AM HAPPY!

What Made Me Feel Happy Today?

_____
_____
_____

I AM THANKFUL!

I Am Thankful For...

_____
_____
_____

TODAY

Date: Sun Mon Tues Weds Thurs Fri Sat ___/___/___

I Feel... ☺ ☺   😐 ☹ ☹

I AM HEALTHY!

What Fruits and Veggies Did I Eat?

_____
_____
_____

How Much Water Did I Drink?

🥛 🥛 🥛 🥛 🥛 🥛 🥛 🥛

I AM HAPPY!

What Made Me Feel Happy Today?

_____
_____
_____

I AM THANKFUL!

I Am Thankful For...

_____
_____
_____

TODAY

Date: Sun Mon Tues Weds Thurs Fri Sat ___/___/___

I Feel... ☺ ☺ 😐 ☹ ☹

I AM HEALTHY!

What Fruits and Veggies Did I Eat?

_____
_____
_____

How Much Water Did I Drink?

🥛 🥛 🥛 🥛 🥛 🥛 🥛 🥛

I AM HAPPY!

What Made Me Feel Happy Today?

_____
_____
_____

I AM THANKFUL!

I Am Thankful For...

_____
_____
_____

TODAY

Date: Sun Mon Tues Weds Thurs Fri Sat ___/___/___

I Feel... 😊 🙂 😐 🙁 ☹️

I AM HEALTHY!

What Fruits and Veggies Did I Eat?

_____
_____
_____

How Much Water Did I Drink?

🥛 🥛 🥛 🥛 🥛 🥛 🥛 🥛

I AM HAPPY!

What Made Me Feel Happy Today?

_____
_____
_____

I AM THANKFUL!

I Am Thankful For...

_____
_____
_____

TODAY

Date: Sun Mon Tues Weds Thurs Fri Sat ___/___/___

I Feel...   ☺   ☺   😐   ☹   ☹

I AM HEALTHY!

What Fruits and Veggies Did I Eat?

_____
_____
_____

How Much Water Did I Drink?

🥛 🥛 🥛 🥛 🥛 🥛 🥛 🥛

I AM HAPPY!

What Made Me Feel Happy Today?

_____
_____
_____

I AM THANKFUL!

I Am Thankful For...

_____
_____
_____

TODAY

Date: Sun Mon Tues Weds Thurs Fri Sat ___/___/___

I Feel... ☺ ☺   😐 ☹ ☹

I AM HEALTHY!

What Fruits and Veggies Did I Eat?

_____
_____
_____

How Much Water Did I Drink?

🥛 🥛 🥛 🥛 🥛 🥛 🥛 🥛

I AM HAPPY!

What Made Me Feel Happy Today?

_____
_____
_____

I AM THANKFUL!

I Am Thankful For...

_____
_____
_____

TODAY

Date: Sun Mon Tues Weds Thurs Fri Sat ___/___/___

I Feel...   ☺   ☺   😐   ☹   ☹

I AM HEALTHY!

What Fruits and Veggies Did I Eat?

_____
_____
_____

How Much Water Did I Drink?

🥤 🥤 🥤 🥤 🥤 🥤 🥤 🥤

I AM HAPPY!

What Made Me Feel Happy Today?

_____
_____
_____

I AM THANKFUL!

I Am Thankful For...

_____
_____
_____

TODAY

Date: Sun Mon Tues Weds Thurs Fri Sat ___/___/___

I Feel... ☺ ☺   😐 ☹ ☹

I AM HEALTHY!

What Fruits and Veggies Did I Eat?

_____
_____
_____

How Much Water Did I Drink?

🥛 🥛 🥛 🥛 🥛 🥛 🥛 🥛

I AM HAPPY!

What Made Me Feel Happy Today?

_____
_____
_____

I AM THANKFUL!

I Am Thankful For...

_____
_____
_____

TODAY

Date: Sun Mon Tues Weds Thurs Fri Sat ___/___/___

I Feel...   ☺   ☺   ☺   ☹   ☹

I AM HEALTHY!

What Fruits and Veggies Did I Eat?

_____
_____
_____

How Much Water Did I Drink?

🥛 🥛 🥛 🥛 🥛 🥛 🥛 🥛

I AM HAPPY!

What Made Me Feel Happy Today?

_____
_____
_____

I AM THANKFUL!

I Am Thankful For...

_____
_____
_____

TODAY

Date: Sun Mon Tues Weds Thurs Fri Sat ___/___/___

I Feel... ☺ ☺ 😐 ☹ ☹

I AM HEALTHY!

What Fruits and Veggies Did I Eat?

_____
_____
_____

How Much Water Did I Drink?

I AM HAPPY!

What Made Me Feel Happy Today?

_____
_____
_____

I AM THANKFUL!

I Am Thankful For...

_____
_____
_____

TODAY

Date: Sun Mon Tues Weds Thurs Fri Sat ___/___/___

I Feel... ☺ ☺ 😐 ☹ ☹

I AM HEALTHY!

What Fruits and Veggies Did I Eat?

_____
_____
_____

How Much Water Did I Drink?

🥛 🥛 🥛 🥛 🥛 🥛 🥛 🥛

I AM HAPPY!

What Made Me Feel Happy Today?

_____
_____
_____

I AM THANKFUL!

I Am Thankful For...

_____
_____
_____

TODAY

Date: Sun Mon Tues Weds Thurs Fri Sat ___/___/___

I Feel... ☺ ☺   😐 ☹ ☹

I AM HEALTHY!

What Fruits and Veggies Did I Eat?

_____
_____
_____

How Much Water Did I Drink?

I AM HAPPY!

What Made Me Feel Happy Today?

_____
_____
_____

I AM THANKFUL!

I Am Thankful For...

_____
_____
_____

TODAY

Date: Sun Mon Tues Weds Thurs Fri Sat ___/___/___

I Feel...   ☺   ☺   😐   ☹   ☹

I AM HEALTHY!

What Fruits and Veggies Did I Eat?

_____
_____
_____

How Much Water Did I Drink?

🥛 🥛 🥛 🥛 🥛 🥛 🥛 🥛

I AM HAPPY!

What Made Me Feel Happy Today?

_____
_____
_____

I AM THANKFUL!

I Am Thankful For...

_____
_____
_____

TODAY

Date: Sun Mon Tues Weds Thurs Fri Sat ___ /___ /___

I Feel... ☺ ☺ 😐 ☹ ☹

I AM HEALTHY!

What Fruits and Veggies Did I Eat?

_____
_____
_____

How Much Water Did I Drink?

🥛 🥛 🥛 🥛 🥛 🥛 🥛 🥛

I AM HAPPY!

What Made Me Feel Happy Today?

_____
_____
_____

I AM THANKFUL!

I Am Thankful For...

_____
_____
_____

TODAY

Date: Sun Mon Tues Weds Thurs Fri Sat ___/___/___

I Feel... 😊 🙂 😐 🙁 ☹️

I AM HEALTHY!

What Fruits and Veggies Did I Eat?

_____
_____
_____

How Much Water Did I Drink?

🥛 🥛 🥛 🥛 🥛 🥛 🥛 🥛

I AM HAPPY!

What Made Me Feel Happy Today?

_____
_____
_____

I AM THANKFUL!

I Am Thankful For...

_____
_____
_____

TODAY

Date: Sun   Mon   Tues   Weds   Thurs   Fri   Sat ___ / ___ / ___

I Feel...   ☺   ☺   ☺   ☹   ☹

I AM HEALTHY!

What Fruits and Veggies Did I Eat?

_____
_____
_____

How Much Water Did I Drink?

I AM HAPPY!

What Made Me Feel Happy Today?

_____
_____
_____

I AM THANKFUL!

I Am Thankful For...

_____
_____
_____

TODAY

Date: Sun Mon Tues Weds Thurs Fri Sat ___/___/___

I Feel... ☺ ☺ 😐 ☹ ☹

I AM HEALTHY!

What Fruits and Veggies Did I Eat?

_____
_____
_____

How Much Water Did I Drink?

🥛 🥛 🥛 🥛 🥛 🥛 🥛 🥛

I AM HAPPY!

What Made Me Feel Happy Today?

_____
_____
_____

I AM THANKFUL!

I Am Thankful For...

_____
_____
_____

TODAY

Date: Sun Mon Tues Weds Thurs Fri Sat ___/___/___

I Feel... ☺ ☺   😐 ☹ ☹

I AM HEALTHY!

What Fruits and Veggies Did I Eat?

_____
_____
_____

How Much Water Did I Drink?

🥤 🥤 🥤 🥤 🥤 🥤 🥤 🥤

I AM HAPPY!

What Made Me Feel Happy Today?

_____
_____
_____

I AM THANKFUL!

I Am Thankful For...

_____
_____
_____

TODAY

Date: Sun Mon Tues Weds Thurs Fri Sat ___/___/___

I Feel... ☺ ☺ ☺ ☹ ☹

I AM HEALTHY!

What Fruits and Veggies Did I Eat?

_____
_____
_____

How Much Water Did I Drink?

🥛 🥛 🥛 🥛 🥛 🥛 🥛 🥛

I AM HAPPY!

What Made Me Feel Happy Today?

_____
_____
_____

I AM THANKFUL!

I Am Thankful For...

_____
_____
_____

TODAY

Date: Sun Mon Tues Weds Thurs Fri Sat ___/___/___

I Feel...   ☺   ☺   😐   ☹   ☹

I AM HEALTHY!

What Fruits and Veggies Did I Eat?

_____
_____
_____

How Much Water Did I Drink?

🥛 🥛 🥛 🥛 🥛 🥛 🥛 🥛

I AM HAPPY!

What Made Me Feel Happy Today?

_____
_____
_____

I AM THANKFUL!

I Am Thankful For...

_____
_____
_____

TODAY

Date: Sun Mon Tues Weds Thurs Fri Sat ___/___/___

I Feel... ☺ ☺ ☻ ☹ ☹

I AM HEALTHY!

What Fruits and Veggies Did I Eat?

_____
_____
_____

How Much Water Did I Drink?

I AM HAPPY!

What Made Me Feel Happy Today?

_____
_____
_____

I AM THANKFUL!

I Am Thankful For...

_____
_____
_____

TODAY

Date: Sun Mon Tues Weds Thurs Fri Sat ___/___/___

I Feel... ☺ ☺ 😐 ☹ ☹

I AM HEALTHY!

What Fruits and Veggies Did I Eat?

_____
_____
_____

How Much Water Did I Drink?

🥛 🥛 🥛 🥛 🥛 🥛 🥛 🥛

I AM HAPPY!

What Made Me Feel Happy Today?

_____
_____
_____

I AM THANKFUL!

I Am Thankful For...

_____
_____
_____

TODAY

Date: Sun Mon Tues Weds Thurs Fri Sat ___/___/___

I Feel... ☺ ☺ 😐 ☹ ☹

I AM HEALTHY!

What Fruits and Veggies Did I Eat?

_____
_____
_____

How Much Water Did I Drink?

🥛 🥛 🥛 🥛 🥛 🥛 🥛 🥛

I AM HAPPY!

What Made Me Feel Happy Today?

_____
_____
_____

I AM THANKFUL!

I Am Thankful For...

_____
_____
_____

TODAY

Date: Sun Mon Tues Weds Thurs Fri Sat ___/___/___

I Feel... ☺ ☺   😐 ☹ ☹

I AM HEALTHY!

What Fruits and Veggies Did I Eat?

_____
_____
_____

How Much Water Did I Drink?

🥛 🥛 🥛 🥛 🥛 🥛 🥛 🥛

I AM HAPPY!

What Made Me Feel Happy Today?

_____
_____
_____

I AM THANKFUL!

I Am Thankful For...

_____
_____
_____

TODAY

Date: Sun Mon Tues Weds Thurs Fri Sat ___/___/___

I Feel...   ☺   ☺   ☺   ☹   ☹

I AM HEALTHY!

What Fruits and Veggies Did I Eat?

_____
_____
_____

How Much Water Did I Drink?

I AM HAPPY!

What Made Me Feel Happy Today?

_____
_____
_____

I AM THANKFUL!

I Am Thankful For...

_____
_____
_____

TODAY

Date: Sun Mon Tues Weds Thurs Fri Sat ___/___/___

I Feel...   ☺   ☺   ☺   ☹   ☹

I AM HEALTHY!

What Fruits and Veggies Did I Eat?

_____
_____
_____

How Much Water Did I Drink?

🥛 🥛 🥛 🥛 🥛 🥛 🥛 🥛

I AM HAPPY!

What Made Me Feel Happy Today?

_____
_____
_____

I AM THANKFUL!

I Am Thankful For...

_____
_____
_____

TODAY

Date: Sun Mon Tues Weds Thurs Fri Sat ___/___/___

I Feel...   ☺   ☺   ☺   ☹   ☹

I AM HEALTHY!

What Fruits and Veggies Did I Eat?
_____
_____
_____

How Much Water Did I Drink?

🥛 🥛 🥛 🥛 🥛 🥛 🥛 🥛

I AM HAPPY!

What Made Me Feel Happy Today?
_____
_____
_____

I AM THANKFUL!

I Am Thankful For...
_____
_____
_____

TODAY

Date: Sun Mon Tues Weds Thurs Fri Sat ___/___/___

I Feel... ☺ ☺   😐 ☹ ☹

I AM HEALTHY!

What Fruits and Veggies Did I Eat?

_____
_____
_____

How Much Water Did I Drink?

I AM HAPPY!

What Made Me Feel Happy Today?

_____
_____
_____

I AM THANKFUL!

I Am Thankful For...

_____
_____
_____

TODAY

Date: Sun Mon Tues Weds Thurs Fri Sat ___/___/___

I Feel... ☺ ☺ 😐 ☹ ☹

I AM HEALTHY!

What Fruits and Veggies Did I Eat?

_____
_____
_____

How Much Water Did I Drink?

🥛 🥛 🥛 🥛 🥛 🥛 🥛 🥛

I AM HAPPY!

What Made Me Feel Happy Today?

_____
_____
_____

I AM THANKFUL!

I Am Thankful For...

_____
_____
_____

TODAY

Date: Sun Mon Tues Weds Thurs Fri Sat ___/___/___

I Feel...   ☺   ☺   😐   ☹   ☹

I AM HEALTHY!

What Fruits and Veggies Did I Eat?

_____
_____
_____

How Much Water Did I Drink?

🥛 🥛 🥛 🥛 🥛 🥛 🥛 🥛

I AM HAPPY!

What Made Me Feel Happy Today?

_____
_____
_____

I AM THANKFUL!

I Am Thankful For...

_____
_____
_____

TODAY

Date: Sun   Mon   Tues   Weds   Thurs   Fri   Sat ___/___/___

I Feel...   😊   🙂   😐   🙁   ☹️

I AM HEALTHY!

What Fruits and Veggies Did I Eat?

_____
_____
_____

How Much Water Did I Drink?

🥛 🥛 🥛 🥛 🥛 🥛 🥛 🥛

I AM HAPPY!

What Made Me Feel Happy Today?

_____
_____
_____

I AM THANKFUL!

I Am Thankful For...

_____
_____
_____

TODAY

Date: Sun Mon Tues Weds Thurs Fri Sat ___/___/___

I Feel... ☺ ☺ 😐 ☹ ☹

I AM HEALTHY!

What Fruits and Veggies Did I Eat?

_____
_____
_____

How Much Water Did I Drink?

🥛 🥛 🥛 🥛 🥛 🥛 🥛 🥛

I AM HAPPY!

What Made Me Feel Happy Today?

_____
_____
_____

I AM THANKFUL!

I Am Thankful For...

_____
_____
_____

TODAY

Date: Sun Mon Tues Weds Thurs Fri Sat ___/___/___

I Feël... ☺ ☺ 😐 🙁 ☹

I AM HEALTHY!

What Fruits and Veggies Did I Eat?

_____
_____
_____

How Much Water Did I Drink?

🥛 🥛 🥛 🥛 🥛 🥛 🥛 🥛

I AM HAPPY!

What Made Me Feel Happy Today?

_____
_____
_____

I AM THANKFUL!

I Am Thankful For...

_____
_____
_____

TODAY

Date: Sun Mon Tues Weds Thurs Fri Sat ___/___/___

I Feel...   ☺   ☺   😐   ☹   ☹

I AM HEALTHY!

What Fruits and Veggies Did I Eat?

_____
_____
_____

How Much Water Did I Drink?

🥛 🥛 🥛 🥛 🥛 🥛 🥛 🥛

I AM HAPPY!

What Made Me Feel Happy Today?

_____
_____
_____

I AM THANKFUL!

I Am Thankful For...

_____
_____
_____

TODAY

Date: Sun Mon Tues Weds Thurs Fri Sat ___/___/___

I Feel...   ☺   🙂   😐   🙁   ☹

I AM HEALTHY!

What Fruits and Veggies Did I Eat?
_____
_____
_____

How Much Water Did I Drink?

🥛 🥛 🥛 🥛 🥛 🥛 🥛 🥛

I AM HAPPY!

What Made Me Feel Happy Today?
_____
_____
_____

I AM THANKFUL!

I Am Thankful For...
_____
_____
_____

TODAY

Date: Sun Mon Tues Weds Thurs Fri Sat ___/___/___

I Feel... ☺ ☺ 😐 ☹ ☹

I AM HEALTHY!

What Fruits and Veggies Did I Eat?

_____
_____
_____

How Much Water Did I Drink?

🥛 🥛 🥛 🥛 🥛 🥛 🥛 🥛

I AM HAPPY!

What Made Me Feel Happy Today?

_____
_____
_____

I AM THANKFUL!

I Am Thankful For...

_____
_____
_____

TODAY

Date: Sun Mon Tues Weds Thurs Fri Sat ___/___/___

I Feel... ☺ ☺ ☺ ☹ ☹

I AM HEALTHY!

What Fruits and Veggies Did I Eat?

_____
_____
_____

How Much Water Did I Drink?

🥛 🥛 🥛 🥛 🥛 🥛 🥛 🥛

I AM HAPPY!

What Made Me Feel Happy Today?

_____
_____
_____

I AM THANKFUL!

I Am Thankful For...

_____
_____
_____

TODAY

Date: Sun Mon Tues Weds Thurs Fri Sat ___ / ___ / ___

I Feel... ☺ ☺ 😐 ☹ ☹

I AM HEALTHY!

What Fruits and Veggies Did I Eat?

_____
_____
_____

How Much Water Did I Drink?

🥛 🥛 🥛 🥛 🥛 🥛 🥛 🥛

I AM HAPPY!

What Made Me Feel Happy Today?

_____
_____
_____

I AM THANKFUL!

I Am Thankful For...

_____
_____
_____

TODAY

Date: Sun   Mon   Tues   Weds   Thurs   Fri   Sat ___/___/___

I Feel...   ☺   ☺   ☺   ☹   ☹

I AM HEALTHY!

What Fruits and Veggies Did I Eat?

_____

_____

_____

How Much Water Did I Drink?

I AM HAPPY!

What Made Me Feel Happy Today?

_____

_____

_____

I AM THANKFUL!

I Am Thankful For...

_____

_____

_____

TODAY

Date: Sun Mon Tues Weds Thurs Fri Sat ___/___/___

I Feel... 😊 🙂 😐 🙁 ☹️

I AM HEALTHY!

What Fruits and Veggies Did I Eat?

_____
_____
_____

How Much Water Did I Drink?

🥛 🥛 🥛 🥛 🥛 🥛 🥛 🥛

I AM HAPPY!

What Made Me Feel Happy Today?

_____
_____
_____

I AM THANKFUL!

I Am Thankful For...

_____
_____
_____

TODAY

Date: Sun Mon Tues Weds Thurs Fri Sat ___/___/___

I Feel... ☺ ☺ ☺ ☹ ☹

I AM HEALTHY!

What Fruits and Veggies Did I Eat?

_____
_____
_____

How Much Water Did I Drink?

🥛 🥛 🥛 🥛 🥛 🥛 🥛 🥛

I AM HAPPY!

What Made Me Feel Happy Today?

_____
_____
_____

I AM THANKFUL!

I Am Thankful For...

_____
_____
_____

TODAY

Date: Sun Mon Tues Weds Thurs Fri Sat ___/___/____

I Feel... ☺ ☺ 😐 ☹ ☹

I AM HEALTHY!

What Fruits and Veggies Did I Eat?

_____
_____
_____

How Much Water Did I Drink?

🥛 🥛 🥛 🥛 🥛 🥛 🥛 🥛

I AM HAPPY!

What Made Me Feel Happy Today?

_____
_____
_____

I AM THANKFUL!

I Am Thankful For...

_____
_____
_____

TODAY

Date: Sun Mon Tues Weds Thurs Fri Sat ___/___/___

I Feel...   ☺   ☺   ☺   ☹   ☹

I AM HEALTHY!

What Fruits and Veggies Did I Eat?

_____
_____
_____

How Much Water Did I Drink?

🥛 🥛 🥛 🥛 🥛 🥛 🥛 🥛

I AM HAPPY!

What Made Me Feel Happy Today?

_____
_____
_____

I AM THANKFUL!

I Am Thankful For...

_____
_____
_____

TODAY

Date: Sun   Mon   Tues   Weds   Thurs   Fri   Sat ___/___/___

I Feel...   ☺   ☺   😐   ☹   ☹

I AM HEALTHY!

What Fruits and Veggies Did I Eat?

_____
_____
_____

How Much Water Did I Drink?

🥛 🥛 🥛 🥛 🥛 🥛 🥛 🥛

I AM HAPPY!

What Made Me Feel Happy Today?

_____
_____
_____

I AM THANKFUL!

I Am Thankful For...

_____
_____
_____

TODAY

Date: Sun Mon Tues Weds Thurs Fri Sat ___/___/___

I Feel... ☺ ☺ 😐 ☹ ☹

I AM HEALTHY!

What Fruits and Veggies Did I Eat?

_____
_____
_____

How Much Water Did I Drink?

🥛 🥛 🥛 🥛 🥛 🥛 🥛 🥛

I AM HAPPY!

What Made Me Feel Happy Today?

_____
_____
_____

I AM THANKFUL!

I Am Thankful For...

_____
_____
_____

TODAY

Date: Sun Mon Tues Weds Thurs Fri Sat ___/___/___

I Feel... ☺ ☺ 😐 ☹ ☹

I AM HEALTHY!

What Fruits and Veggies Did I Eat?

_____
_____
_____

How Much Water Did I Drink?

🥛 🥛 🥛 🥛 🥛 🥛 🥛 🥛

I AM HAPPY!

What Made Me Feel Happy Today?

_____
_____
_____

I AM THANKFUL!

I Am Thankful For...

_____
_____
_____

TODAY

Date: Sun Mon Tues Weds Thurs Fri Sat ___/___/___

I Feel... ☺ ☺ ☺ ☹ ☹

I AM HEALTHY!

What Fruits and Veggies Did I Eat?

_____
_____
_____

How Much Water Did I Drink?

🥛 🥛 🥛 🥛 🥛 🥛 🥛 🥛

I AM HAPPY!

What Made Me Feel Happy Today?

_____
_____
_____

I AM THANKFUL!

I Am Thankful For...

_____
_____
_____

TODAY

Date: Sun Mon Tues Weds Thurs Fri Sat ___/___/___

I Feel...   ☺   ☺   ☺   ☹   ☹

I AM HEALTHY!

What Fruits and Veggies Did I Eat?

_____
_____
_____

How Much Water Did I Drink?

🥛 🥛 🥛 🥛 🥛 🥛 🥛 🥛

I AM HAPPY!

What Made Me Feel Happy Today?

_____
_____
_____

I AM THANKFUL!

I Am Thankful For...

_____
_____
_____

TODAY

Date: Sun Mon Tues Weds Thurs Fri Sat ___/___/___

I Feel...   ☺   ☺   😐   ☹   ☹

I AM HEALTHY!

What Fruits and Veggies Did I Eat?

_____

_____

_____

How Much Water Did I Drink?

🥛 🥛 🥛 🥛 🥛 🥛 🥛 🥛

I AM HAPPY!

What Made Me Feel Happy Today?

_____

_____

_____

I AM THANKFUL!

I Am Thankful For...

_____

_____

_____

TODAY

Date: Sun Mon Tues Weds Thurs Fri Sat ___/___/___

I Feel... ☺   ☺   😐   ☹   ☹

I AM HEALTHY!

What Fruits and Veggies Did I Eat?

_____
_____
_____

How Much Water Did I Drink?

🥛 🥛 🥛 🥛 🥛 🥛 🥛 🥛

I AM HAPPY!

What Made Me Feel Happy Today?

_____
_____
_____

I AM THANKFUL!

I Am Thankful For...

_____
_____
_____

TODAY

Date: Sun Mon Tues Weds Thurs Fri Sat ___/___/___

I Feel... ☺   ☺   ☺   ☹   ☹

I AM HEALTHY!

What Fruits and Veggies Did I Eat?

_____

_____

_____

How Much Water Did I Drink?

🥛 🥛 🥛 🥛 🥛 🥛 🥛 🥛

I AM HAPPY!

What Made Me Feel Happy Today?

_____

_____

_____

I AM THANKFUL!

I Am Thankful For...

_____

_____

_____

TODAY

Date: Sun   Mon   Tues   Weds   Thurs   Fri   Sat ___/___/___

I Feel...   ☺   ☺   ☺   ☹   ☹

I AM HEALTHY!

What Fruits and Veggies Did I Eat?

_____
_____
_____

How Much Water Did I Drink?

🥛 🥛 🥛 🥛 🥛 🥛 🥛 🥛

I AM HAPPY!

What Made Me Feel Happy Today?

_____
_____
_____

I AM THANKFUL!

I Am Thankful For...

_____
_____
_____

TODAY

Date: Sun Mon Tues Weds Thurs Fri Sat ___/___/___

I Feel... ☺ ☺ 😐 ☹ ☹

I AM HEALTHY!

What Fruits and Veggies Did I Eat?

_____
_____
_____

How Much Water Did I Drink?

🥛 🥛 🥛 🥛 🥛 🥛 🥛 🥛

I AM HAPPY!

What Made Me Feel Happy Today?

_____
_____
_____

I AM THANKFUL!

I Am Thankful For...

_____
_____
_____

TODAY

Date: Sun Mon Tues Weds Thurs Fri Sat ___/___/___

I Feel... 😊 🙂 😐 🙁 ☹️

I AM HEALTHY!

What Fruits and Veggies Did I Eat?

_____
_____
_____

How Much Water Did I Drink?

I AM HAPPY!

What Made Me Feel Happy Today?

_____
_____
_____

I AM THANKFUL!

I Am Thankful For...

_____
_____
_____

TODAY

Date: Sun Mon Tues Weds Thurs Fri Sat ___/___/___

I Feel... ☺ ☺   😐 ☹ ☹

I AM HEALTHY!

What Fruits and Veggies Did I Eat?

_____
_____
_____

How Much Water Did I Drink?

🥛 🥛 🥛 🥛 🥛 🥛 🥛 🥛

I AM HAPPY!

What Made Me Feel Happy Today?

_____
_____
_____

I AM THANKFUL!

I Am Thankful For...

_____
_____
_____

TODAY

Date: Sun Mon Tues Weds Thurs Fri Sat ___ /___ /___

I Feel... ☺ ☺ 😐 ☹ ☹

I AM HEALTHY!

What Fruits and Veggies Did I Eat?

_____
_____
_____

How Much Water Did I Drink?

🥛 🥛 🥛 🥛 🥛 🥛 🥛 🥛

I AM HAPPY!

What Made Me Feel Happy Today?

_____
_____
_____

I AM THANKFUL!

I Am Thankful For...

_____
_____
_____

TODAY

Date: Sun Mon Tues Weds Thurs Fri Sat ___/___/___

I Feel... ☺ ☺ ☺ ☹ ☹

I AM HEALTHY!

What Fruits and Veggies Did I Eat?

How Much Water Did I Drink?

I AM HAPPY!

What Made Me Feel Happy Today?

I AM THANKFUL!

I Am Thankful For...

TODAY

Date: Sun Mon Tues Weds Thurs Fri Sat ___/___/___

I Feel... ☺   ☺   ☺   ☹   ☹

I AM HEALTHY!

What Fruits and Veggies Did I Eat?

_____
_____
_____

How Much Water Did I Drink?

🥛 🥛 🥛 🥛 🥛 🥛 🥛 🥛

I AM HAPPY!

What Made Me Feel Happy Today?

_____
_____
_____

I AM THANKFUL!

I Am Thankful For...

_____
_____
_____

TODAY

Date: Sun Mon Tues Weds Thurs Fri Sat ___/___/___

I Feel... ☺ ☺   😐 ☹ ☹

I AM HEALTHY!

What Fruits and Veggies Did I Eat?

_____
_____
_____

How Much Water Did I Drink?

🥛 🥛 🥛 🥛 🥛 🥛 🥛 🥛

I AM HAPPY!

What Made Me Feel Happy Today?

_____
_____
_____

I AM THANKFUL!

I Am Thankful For...

_____
_____
_____

TODAY

Date: Sun Mon Tues Weds Thurs Fri Sat ___/___/___

I Feël... 😊 🙂 😐 🙁 ☹️

I AM HEALTHY!

What Fruits and Veggies Did I Eat?
_____
_____
_____

How Much Water Did I Drink?

I AM HAPPY!

What Made Me Feel Happy Today?
_____
_____
_____

I AM THANKFUL!

I Am Thankful For...
_____
_____
_____

TODAY

Date: Sun Mon Tues Weds Thurs Fri Sat ___/___/___

I Feel... ☺ ☺   😐 ☹ ☹

I AM HEALTHY!

What Fruits and Veggies Did I Eat?

_____
_____
_____

How Much Water Did I Drink?

🥛 🥛 🥛 🥛 🥛 🥛 🥛 🥛

I AM HAPPY!

What Made Me Feel Happy Today?

_____
_____
_____

I AM THANKFUL!

I Am Thankful For...

_____
_____
_____

TODAY

Date: Sun Mon Tues Weds Thurs Fri Sat ___/___/___

I Feel... ☺ ☺ 😐 ☹ ☹

I AM HEALTHY!

What Fruits and Veggies Did I Eat?

_____
_____
_____

How Much Water Did I Drink?

🥛 🥛 🥛 🥛 🥛 🥛 🥛 🥛

I AM HAPPY!

What Made Me Feel Happy Today?

_____
_____
_____

I AM THANKFUL!

I Am Thankful For...

_____
_____
_____

TODAY

Date: Sun Mon Tues Weds Thurs Fri Sat ___/___/___

I Feel... ☺ ☺ ☺ ☹ ☹

I AM HEALTHY!

What Fruits and Veggies Did I Eat?

_____
_____
_____

How Much Water Did I Drink?

I AM HAPPY!

What Made Me Feel Happy Today?

_____
_____
_____

I AM THANKFUL!

I Am Thankful For...

_____
_____
_____

TODAY

Date: Sun   Mon   Tues   Weds   Thurs   Fri   Sat ___/___/___

I Feel...   ☺   ☺   😐   ☹   ☹

I AM HEALTHY!

What Fruits and Veggies Did I Eat?

_____
_____
_____

How Much Water Did I Drink?

🥛 🥛 🥛 🥛 🥛 🥛 🥛 🥛

I AM HAPPY!

What Made Me Feel Happy Today?

_____
_____
_____

I AM THANKFUL!

I Am Thankful For...

_____
_____
_____

TODAY

Date: Sun Mon Tues Weds Thurs Fri Sat ___/___/___

I Feël...   ☺   ☺   ☺   ☹   ☹

I AM HEALTHY!

What Fruits and Veggies Did I Eat?

_____
_____
_____

How Much Water Did I Drink?

🥛 🥛 🥛 🥛 🥛 🥛 🥛 🥛

I AM HAPPY!

What Made Me Feel Happy Today?

_____
_____
_____

I AM THANKFUL!

I Am Thankful For...

_____
_____
_____

TODAY

Date: Sun Mon Tues Weds Thurs Fri Sat ___/___/___

I Feel... ☺ ☺ 😐 ☹ ☹

I AM HEALTHY!

What Fruits and Veggies Did I Eat?

_____
_____
_____

How Much Water Did I Drink?

🥛 🥛 🥛 🥛 🥛 🥛 🥛 🥛

I AM HAPPY!

What Made Me Feel Happy Today?

_____
_____
_____

I AM THANKFUL!

I Am Thankful For...

_____
_____
_____

TODAY

Date: Sun Mon Tues Weds Thurs Fri Sat ___/___/___

I Feel... ☺ ☺   😐 ☹ ☹

I AM HEALTHY!

What Fruits and Veggies Did I Eat?

_____
_____
_____

How Much Water Did I Drink?

🥛 🥛 🥛 🥛 🥛 🥛 🥛 🥛

I AM HAPPY!

What Made Me Feel Happy Today?

_____
_____
_____

I AM THANKFUL!

I Am Thankful For...

_____
_____
_____

TODAY

Date: Sun Mon Tues Weds Thurs Fri Sat ___/___/___

I Feel...   ☺   ☺   ☺   ☹   ☹

I AM HEALTHY!

What Fruits and Veggies Did I Eat?

_____
_____
_____

How Much Water Did I Drink?

I AM HAPPY!

What Made Me Feel Happy Today?

_____
_____
_____

I AM THANKFUL!

I Am Thankful For...

_____
_____
_____

TODAY

Date: Sun Mon Tues Weds Thurs Fri Sat ___/___/___

I Feel... ☺ ☺ ☺ ☹ ☹

I AM HEALTHY!

What Fruits and Veggies Did I Eat?

_____
_____
_____

How Much Water Did I Drink?

I AM HAPPY!

What Made Me Feel Happy Today?

_____
_____
_____

I AM THANKFUL!

I Am Thankful For...

_____
_____
_____

TODAY

Date: Sun Mon Tues Weds Thurs Fri Sat ___/___/___

I Feel... ☺ ☺ 😐 ☹ ☹

I AM HEALTHY!

What Fruits and Veggies Did I Eat?

_____
_____
_____

How Much Water Did I Drink?

🥛 🥛 🥛 🥛 🥛 🥛 🥛 🥛

I AM HAPPY!

What Made Me Feel Happy Today?

_____
_____
_____

I AM THANKFUL!

I Am Thankful For...

_____
_____
_____

TODAY

Date: Sun Mon Tues Weds Thurs Fri Sat ___/___/___

I Feel... ☺ ☺ 😐 ☹ ☹

I AM HEALTHY!

What Fruits and Veggies Did I Eat?

_____
_____
_____

How Much Water Did I Drink?

🥛 🥛 🥛 🥛 🥛 🥛 🥛 🥛

I AM HAPPY!

What Made Me Feel Happy Today?

_____
_____
_____

I AM THANKFUL!

I Am Thankful For...

_____
_____
_____

TODAY

Date: Sun Mon Tues Weds Thurs Fri Sat ___/___/___

I Feel... ☺ ☺ 😐 ☹ ☹

I AM HEALTHY!

What Fruits and Veggies Did I Eat?
_____
_____
_____

How Much Water Did I Drink?

🥛 🥛 🥛 🥛 🥛 🥛 🥛 🥛

I AM HAPPY!

What Made Me Feel Happy Today?
_____
_____
_____

I AM THANKFUL!

I Am Thankful For...
_____
_____
_____

TODAY

Date: Sun Mon Tues Weds Thurs Fri Sat ___/___/___

I Feel... 😊 🙂 😐 🙁 ☹️

I AM HEALTHY!

What Fruits and Veggies Did I Eat?

_____
_____
_____

How Much Water Did I Drink?

🥛 🥛 🥛 🥛 🥛 🥛 🥛 🥛

I AM HAPPY!

What Made Me Feel Happy Today?

_____
_____
_____

I AM THANKFUL!

I Am Thankful For...

_____
_____
_____

TODAY

Date: Sun Mon Tues Weds Thurs Fri Sat ___/___/___

I Feel...   ☺   ☺   😐   ☹   ☹

I AM HEALTHY!

What Fruits and Veggies Did I Eat?

_____
_____
_____

How Much Water Did I Drink?

🥛 🥛 🥛 🥛 🥛 🥛 🥛 🥛

I AM HAPPY!

What Made Me Feel Happy Today?

_____
_____
_____

I AM THANKFUL!

I Am Thankful For...

_____
_____
_____

TODAY

Date: Sun Mon Tues Weds Thurs Fri Sat ___/___/___

I Feel... 😊   🙂   😐   🙁   ☹️

I AM HEALTHY!

What Fruits and Veggies Did I Eat?

_____
_____
_____

How Much Water Did I Drink?

🥛 🥛 🥛 🥛 🥛 🥛 🥛 🥛

I AM HAPPY!

What Made Me Feel Happy Today?

_____
_____
_____

I AM THANKFUL!

I Am Thankful For...

_____
_____
_____

www.ingramcontent.com/pod-product-compliance
Lightning Source LLC
Chambersburg PA
CBHW071116030426
42336CB00013BA/2117